TEA CLEANSE

By Julia Bond

Copyright © 2017 by Julia Bond

Disclaimer and Terms of Use: The Author and Publisher has strived to be as accurate and complete as possible in the creation of this book, notwithstanding the fact that he does not warrant or represent at any time that the contents within are accurate due to the rapidly changing nature of the Internet. While all attempts have been made to verify information provided in this publication, the Author and Publisher assumes no responsibility for errors, omissions, or contrary interpretation of the subject matter herein.

Any perceived slights of specific persons, peoples, or organizations are unintentional. In practical advice books, like anything else in life, there are no guarantees of results. Readers are cautioned to rely on their own judgment about their individual circumstances and act accordingly.

This book is not intended for use as a source of legal, medical, business, accounting or financial advice. All readers are advised to seek services of competent professionals in the legal, medical, business, accounting, and finance fields.

TABLE OF CONTENTS

INTRODUCTION

Before investing in a 200$ tea set, or booking a flight to China to experience an authentic tea house, here's some basic tea history and knowledge to get your feet wet:

Tea is made when the leaves of the plant Camella sinensis are boiled in water. Basically, the leaves are boiled with water in a tea infuser (fancy word for teapot), and removed again in several minutes.

Camella sinensis plant takes a while to grow; it takes around three years before a new tea plant to be ready for harvesting. This isn't like growing tomatoes! When harvesting, only the top 1-2 inches of the plant are cut and used for tea. The harvested leaves and seed are known as flushes. The tea is then processed. Exactly how the tea gets processed depends what type of tea you desire (shown below).

In general, tea quality depends on two factors. The first is the height at which the plant is grown. The Traditional Chinese Tea Cultivation and Studies group concluded that tea plants grown at an altitude of around 1,500 meters, or 4,900 feet, tend to produce a better flavor. The second factor is the size of the tea leaves themselves. The smaller a tea leaf, the higher the quality (and cost) of the tea. Less really is more!

The earliest mention of tea in the Orient dates back to an ancient Chinese myth in 2737 b.c. The Chinese Emperor Shennog was boiling a large pot of water (who knows why) when tea leaves blew into the pot. After tasting this concoction (ol' Shennog was an adventurous one), he immediately fell in love with his discovery. He claimed the beverage was invigorating and promoted a sense of well-being. The popularity of tea steadily during the Han Dynasty (206b.c. - 220a.d.) in China, and by the 8th century the Chinese writer Lu Yu created the first book on the subject of tea. It was called the Ch'a Ching, translated as 'Tea Classic'.

Around this time, tea was introduced to Japan though Buddhist monks who came to China to study. These monks brought tea leaves back to their home island, where demand for tea rose faster than a Chinese firework! From there, tea was introduced to India, Britan, and other parts of the world. However, it is in the Orient that tea has its true roots.

THE MANY DIFFERENT TYPES OF TEA

GREEN TEA

This kind of tea is extremely popular and it contains catechins, which is an antioxidant.

A lot of people drink green tea because of the potential benefits, which includes playing a role in decreasing your risk of getting cardiovascular disease.

It is also worth pointing out that some people drink green tea because they believe that you can lose weight by drinking green tea.

One of the reasons why green tea is thought to help people lose weight is because it boosts the metabolic rate.

BLACK

Black is one of the most commonly drank teas, and it does contain quite a bit of caffeine, at least when compare to other types of tea.

There are two antioxidants that are found in black tea, and these two have been known to lower cholesterol levels.

Also, if you drink three or more cups of this kind of tea on a daily basis, then you could end up cutting your risk of stroke by up to 21 percent.

WHITE

If you are looking for a really healthy tea, then look no further than white tea. White tea contains catechins, just like green tea. Consuming white tea on a regular basis may even reduce the risk of having a recurrence of cancer in breast cancer survivors.

Asides from that, this kind is the purest of all teas, and it is the least processed of them all.

White tea is not fermented, and the leaves that are used to make it are dried naturally, usually via sun drying or steaming methods.

Don't worry about whether or not this tea has a plain taste to it because it does have a slight sweetness to it, so you will love drinking it.

OOLONG

This tea is often served in Chinese restaurants, and it is known being very flavorful, so if you want to drink a tea with a sweet taste to it, then Oolong tea is for you.

You should know that Oolong tea is expensive, and most Oolongs come from Taiwan and it is only semi-fermented. Many drinkers prefer to drink it without milk, lemon or sugar.

This isn't because they don't like sugar, lemon or milk, it is because this kind of tea has a very delicate flavor.

PU ERH

Pu Erh has a very rich and smooth taste to it, and the aging process lasts for a longtime. Sometimes the process can take years to complete, or it can take as little as a few months.

As for what the health benefits are, there are a number of them, and this includes playing a role in lowering your cholesterol levels, as well as help your digestion.

One of the things that make this tea stand out from other teas is that it is fermented twice, and then it is matured.

A lot of people do drink Pu Erh Tea for pleasure, but there are also many people who drink it for medicinal purposes.

FLAVORED

People brew tea from various things, including berries, onions, peach leaves and orange peels. Certain types of flowers are also used for tea. Herbs, spices and oils are often used too.

If you are looking for teas that have unique tastes to it, or you just want tea with some strong flavor to it, then you will want to get your hands on some flavored tea.

BLENDS

Blends are teas that are not from a single lineage, hence the name. Teas that fall under this category of tea has been made with other different types of teas.

Each tea comes with their own benefits; although most of their benefits may be similar. For the most part, depending on what type of tea it is, it can improve brain functions, decrease the chance of cancer, cardiovascular diseases and diabetes, relief stress, strengthen bones, aid weight loss, improve skin, aid digestion, relief cramps and spasms, and act as a sleep aid. That means, drinking tea can make one smarter in some ways. Drinking tea is beneficial for many organs, especially the heart. It can help others relax, not stress, and not go through depression. Less caffeine in tea means less sugar and a lesser change to get type 2 diabetes.

For best results, each type of tea should be prepared differently as well. The basic types of tea are:

White: Is wilted, and unoxidized.

Boiled at 65 to 70 °C (149 to 158 °F) for 1-2 minutes.

Yellow: Is unwilted and unoxidized, and left to turn a yellow color.

Boiled at 70 to 75 °C (158 to 167 °F) for 1-2 minutes.

Green: Is unwilted and unoxidized.

Boiled at 75 to 80 °C (167 to 176 °F) for 1-2 minutes.

Oolong: Is wilted and brusied; partially oxidized.

Boiled at 80 to 85 °C (176 to 185 °F) for 2-3 minutes.

Black: Is wilted, often crushed, and completely oxidized.

Boiled at 99 °C (210 °F) for 2-3 minutes.

Herbal:

Boiled at 99 °C (210 °F) for 3-6 minutes.

CHAPTER 1:
LOSS WEIGHT WITH TEA

Proper diet and exercise and even counting calories are still the long-standing approaches to weight loss problems. But the issue seems to have reached a point where pharmaceutical products had to be developed to directly treat abnormal weight gain. Some of the more popular diet pills available today are designed to either make you less able to digest fat content in food or suppress your appetite. Fortunately there's a natural alternative to taking a pill or two. You can build the habit of drinking a cup of tea two to three times a day. Tea works better than diet pills because it simultaneously provides the anti-obesity mechanisms that such pills singularly offer. So with every cup you're already enabling your body to deal with fats and curb your appetite. That's just for weight control, one set of benefits among a host of others that green tea delivers.

LESSEN FAT DIGESTION

There's nothing wrong with fats per se. This macronutrient along with carbohydrates is after all one of the fuel sources that your body breaks down and processes to produce energy. It's when too much is consumed, stored and left unused that abnormal weight gain and the problems that come with it happen. Lipases are the type of enzymes that, among other functions, play a role in metabolizing fats. Gastric and pancreatic lipases are the ones that directly perform this operation. These are also the lipases that the catechins in green tea inhibit. One in vitro study was able to show how a green tree extract containing 25% of the catechins was able to reduce the gastric lipase breakdown of fats by around 96% and partially do the same for pancreatic lipase at 66%. Why is this important for someone trying to control his or her weight? When fats in food aren't properly broken down in the digestive system, they can't get absorbed and just pass through. That means less additional burden to what may already be abundant stores of fat tissue.

Follow up research on the study mentioned was done, this time with human participants. The subjects were described as moderately obese. After three months of taking the same green tea extract, they experienced a 4.6 % reduction in body weight and their waists were smaller by 4.48 %. In the in vitro study mentioned earlier, it only took 60 mg of the green tea extract formulated with 25% catechins to produce the significant gastric fat breakdown reduction. Imagine what weight loss effects can be achieved by ingesting more concentrated forms. Eating as well as drinking green tea can actually provide more of these beneficial substances.

CURB APPETITE

The feeling of satiety is brought about by a complex process that involves the interaction of hormones, peptides, and other chemicals that send and receive nerve signals. As it turns out, the substances in green tea seem to be able to affect this process. Researchers on a study that was investigating the impact of green tea on glucose, insulin and satiety levels were somewhat surprised that the participants who took in green tea along with a meal felt fuller and had no desire to eat more.

After eliminating other possible causes, they theorized that the green tea catechins enabled the neurotransmitter called norepinephrine to act longer on the brain and establish the feeling of satiety. The reason is that the catechins blocked the enzyme (catechol-o-methyl-transferase) that breaks down the neurotransmitter. Lessening the digestion of fat and suppressing appetite is actually just two of the weight loss benefits that green tea can offer.

USE GREEN TEA TO INCREASE EXERCISE ENDURANCE

Exercise is a way of life for many people, but so is tiring quickly. In order to keep fit and healthy it's essential that regular exercise is undertaken, but to prevent the dreaded burn out there's a surprising little helper – green tea. Among the many other benefits of green tea, it can be used to: increase exercise endurance, improve performance, and prolong workout sessions. Studies are confirming this fact as well, with one having been conducted by Murase et al. The researchers wanted to look at the effects of green tea catechins in relation to endurance, fat oxidization and energy metabolism, using mice as subjects. Over a 10-week period the mice were given different levels of green tea extract and then had to swim to exhaustion, with results showing that the mice that were fed higher doses of green tea could swim for 8-24% longer. This shows the increased endurance effects of green tea, with researchers also finding that higher doses led to reduced respiratory quotients and increased levels of fat oxidization. So, as well as being a great way to increase exercise endurance, the results also indicate that green tea can be good for overall fitness and fat loss. But why is that? A lot of people think it's the caffeine content that keeps us going, and while that could quite possibly play a part it seems that there's a bit more to it than that. As with a lot of the benefits of green tea, it largely comes down to the antioxidants contained within it. The above study even focused part of its research on the effects of epigallocatechin gallate, a primary antioxidant of green, finding that the endurance-enhancing effects of green tea were largely down to this one catechin. Don't be put off by the fact that the study was conducted on mice. Murase estimates that for an athlete to see the same effects as was apparent in the study, they'd have to drink just four cups of green tea a day. And, it's also worth noting that a single high dose of green tea catechins won't do the trick. The study showed that this didn't affect performance at all. Rather, it's the long-term consumption of green tea that will have the most effect. As it only requires four cups a day, it's hardly a major lifestyle inconvenience.

So, green tea really can be used to increase exercise endurance. It would be a great dietary addition for athletes who want to improve their performance, or even for novices who want to get started with a bit of a helping hand. Either way, green tea is incredibly beneficial. As it has plenty of other health benefits, it's a great addition to anyone's diet with numerous studies confirming it.

THE EFFECTS OF GREEN TEA ON WEIGHT LOSS

Green tea has long been thought to have a number of health benefits, and the fact that it can even be used as a way to help weight loss has many dieters clamoring to get their hands on it. But can green tea live up to its claims of being a useful weight loss aide? That's what scientists are trying to find out. So far, studies into the effects that green tea can have on weight loss seem to be promising. There are a lot of studies indicating that just adding green tea into our diet can have a significant impact on our ability to lose weight, with one being published in the American Journal of Clinical Nutrition in 2005. In the study, conducted in Tokyo by Nagao et al, participants were given 690 mg catechins (a type of antioxidant found in green tea) per day. After 12 weeks participants displayed significantly reduced levels of body fat, with researchers concluding that daily consumption of green tea could therefore be beneficial in the fight to lose weight and in the prevention of obesity.

Other studies offer similar findings. One study, which was conducted in Japan by Shimotoyodome et al in 2005, used mice as test subjects and divided them into five groups. Each were fed a high-fat diet with one group receiving daily green tea extract, another one green tea extract plus exercise, and the rest being given varying levels of exercise but no green tea. The results were quite astounding despite the high-fat diet, the mice that had the green tea extract exhibited a 47% reduction in weight gain and those who had the extract plus exercise showed a massive 89% reduction. Although this study was conducted with mice, it wouldn't be so hard to envisage the same type of effects being possible with humans, as shown in other studies. This indicates that just drinking green tea can help to prevent us from gaining weight even if we don't alter our diet in any other way. Of course eating a healthy diet as well would be even more beneficial! So, what could be causing these weight loss effects? A number of theories are being offered, with just one of them being the ability of green tea to raise our metabolism. Green tea contains caffeine, and drinking moderate amounts of caffeine can increase our metabolism and thus our ability to burn more fat. The caffeine content also means that we'll be more energetic, which, subsequently, can lead to increased levels of activity and as such increased levels of calorie burning.

But is it just the level of caffeine in green tea that means we burn more energy? Actually, there's more to it than that. In a study conducted by the Department of Physiology at the University of Geneva in 1999, participants were randomly given green tea extract plus caffeine, just caffeine or a placebo on different days. The results showed that the participants expended more energy and burned far more calories on the days that they were given green tea plus caffeine than they did on any other days, indicating that there are other factors in green tea besides its caffeine content that give rise to its ability to help us lose weight and expend energy. It could be down to antioxidants instead. The antioxidants contained in green tea, particularly catechins, raise our metabolism by encouraging a process known as thermogenesis – the raising of our body temperature leading to an increase in the number of calories being burned – meaning that this could also have an impact in the ability of green tea to reduce weight. So, green tea really can be beneficial in our attempts to lose weight. Researchers suggest that drinking around 5-6 cups of green tea per day can have the most benefit, and if you substitute your regular tea or coffee for green tea then you're sure to notice the effects. Make sure to give green tea a go and see if it can help you in your weight loss quest.

CHAPTER 2:
HEALTH BENEFITS OF TEA

Put down those saucer cups and get chugging — tea is officially awesome for your health. But before loading up on Red Zinger, make sure that your "tea" is actually tea. Real tea is derived from a particular plant (Camellia sinensis) and includes only four varieties: green, black, white, and oolong. Anything else (like herbal "tea") is an infusion of a different plant and isn't technically tea.

But what real tea lacks in variety, it makes up for with some serious health benefits. Researchers attribute tea's health properties to polyphenols (a type of antioxidant) and phytochemicals. Though most studies have focused on the better-known green and black teas, white and oolong also bring benefits to the table. Read on to find out why coffee's little cousin rocks your health.

Tea has been an important beverage for thousands of years and has been a huge part of culture in countries around the world, forming major parts of ceremonies, trade routes and even starting revolutions. But tea isn't just appreciated for its good taste and worldwide appeal, it also offers numerous health benefits. Here are a few health conscious reasons you should add a cup of tea to your daily routine.

OVERALL HEALTH

Tea can be beneficial to your whole body as you can see from these great effects.

Tea contains antioxidants. Antioxidants can help slow down aging and help your cells to regenerate and repair. Teas of all varieties contain high levels of antioxidant polyphenols that can help keep your body healthier and some studies suggest even ward of some cancers.

Tea has less caffeine than coffee. While there are some potential health benefits to consuming moderate amounts of caffeine, drinking loads of it is hard on your heart and other organs. Tea can provide the pick me up of coffee but without the high levels of caffeine making you less jittery and helping you get to sleep when you want.

Tea helps keep you hydrated. Conventional wisdom held that caffeinated beverages actually dehydrated you more than they hydrated you. Recent research has shown, however, that caffeine doesn't make a difference unless you consume more than 5 to 6 cups at a time. Tea has been shown to actually be more healthy for you than water alone in some cases because it hydrates while providing antioxidants.

MENTAL HEALTH

Boost your brain and mental state with these benefits of tea.

Tea can create a calmer but more alert state of mind. Studies have shown that the amino acid L-theanine found in the tea plant alters the attention networks in the brain and can have demonstrable effects on the brain waves. More simply, tea can help you relax and concentrate more fully on tasks.

Tea lowers the chance of having cognitive impairment. Research on Japanese adults who consumed at least 2 cups of green tea daily found that those individuals had cut their risk of cognitive impairment by half.

Tea lowers stress hormone levels. Black tea has been shown to reduce the effects of a stressful event. Participants in a study experienced a 20% drop in cortisol, a stress hormone, after drinking 4 cups of tea daily for one month.

Tea eases irritability, headaches, nervous tension and insomnia. Red tea, also known as rooibos, is an herbal tea that originated in Africa. It has been show to have many relaxing effects that help reduce a wide range of irritations and inflammations on the body.

Tea can cause a temporary increase in short term memory. Not feeling on your game today? Try drinking some tea. The caffeine it contains may give you the boost you need to improve your memory, at least for a few hours.

HEART AND OTHER ORGANS

Help protect your heart and other organs with these beneficial effects of tea.

Tea may reduce your risk of heart attack and stroke. Tea helps to prevent the formation of dangerous blood clots which are very often the cause of heart attacks and strokes. Some studies have even found that black tea drinkers were at a 70 percent lower risk of having a fatal heart attack.

Tea protects your bones. You don't have to put milk in your tea for it to help out your bones. Studies have shown that regular tea drinkers have stronger bones than those of non tea drinkers, even when other variables were adjusted for. Scientists have theorized it may be a benefit of the phytochemicals in tea.

Tea may protect against heart disease. While more studies are needed for conclusive evidence, it has been suggested that regular consumption of green and black tea leads to a significant reduction in the risk of heart disease related heart attacks.

Tea can help lower cholesterol.A recent study in China has shown that the combination of a low-fat diet and tea produced on average a 16% drop in bad cholesterol over 12 weeks when compared to a control group simply on a low-fat diet. If you're struggling to get your cholesterol under control, try adding tea to your diet to see if it helps.

Tea can help lower blood pressure. Drinking only half a cup of green or oolong tea a day could reduce your risk of high blood pressure by up to 50% and those that drink more can even further reduce their risk, even if they have additional risk factors.

Tea aids in digestion. Tea has been used in China for thousands of years as an after-meal digestive aid and it can help you as well due to the high levels of tannins it contains.

Tea helps inhibit intestinal inflammation. The polyphenols in green tea have been shown to have an effect on the intestinal inflammation caused by conditions like Irritable Bowel Syndrome allowing sufferers more comfort from a natural remedy.

Tea can reduce stomach cramps. Properties of red tea cause it to acts as anti-spasmodic agent and allowing it to aid in the relief of stomach cramps or even colic in infants.

FITNESS AND APPEARANCE

Tea can not only help you feel good but look good too.

Tea helps protect your smile. While the stereotype of the tea-drinking Brits with horrible teeth may make you think otherwise, tea actually contains fluoride and tannins, both of which help reduce plaque buildup and tooth decay. Combined with a good dental hygiene regimen, this could keep your teeth healthier for longer.

Tea is calorie-free. Tea itself has no calories unless you choose to add sweeteners or milk, making it a satisfying, low-cal way to wake up and maybe even shed a few pounds.

Tea increases your metabolism. Is a slow metabolic rate keeping you from losing the weight you want? Some studies suggest that green tea may be able to boost your metabolic rate slightly, allowing you to burn an additional 70-80 calories a day. While this may not seem like much, over time it could add up.

Tea helps keep your skin acne-free. The antioxidants in green tea may have an effect on acne, and in some cases have been shown to work as well as a 4% solution of the much more harsh benzoyl peroxide.

Tea can help bad breath. A study at the University of Chicago has suggested that the polyphenols in tea can help to keep the bacteria that causes bad breath in check.

ILLNESS AND DISEASE

Check out these benefits of tea which may help prevent you from getting sick.

Tea strengthens your immune defenses. You may want to drink a cup of tea the next time a cold is going around your office. A recent study compared the immune activity in coffee drinkers to that of tea drinkers and found it to be much higher (up to five times) in those that chose tea. While it's no guarantee against a cold, it sure couldn't hurt.

Tea protects against cancer. While the exact types of cancer tea protects against are debated, recent research has suggested that lung, prostate and breast cancer see the biggest drop when green tea is consumed regularly. Again, there is no surefire way to prevent getting cancer, but having a cup of tea a day may is definitely worth the preventative benefits.

Tea can help prevent arthritis. Research suggests that older women who are tea drinkers are 60 percent less likely to develop rheumatoid arthritis than those who do not drink tea. The same effect has not been measured in older males, however, but additional studies may prove otherwise.

Tea can help fight the flu. Black tea may bolster your efforts to fight the flu as participants in a study who gargled with a black tea extract solution twice daily where more immune to the flu virus than those who didn't.

Tea helps fight infection. Tea contains chemicals called alkylamine antigens which act similarly to some tumor cells and bacteria, boosting the body's immune response. It has even been shown to have an effect on severe infections like sepsis.

Tea may reduce the risk of Parkinson's Disease. New studies are suggesting that regular tea consumption may help protect the body from developing this neurological disorder.

Tea can prevent food poisoning. Catechin, one of the bitter ingredients found in green tea has been shown to effectively kill the bacteria which cause food poisoning and minimize the effects of the toxins that are produced by those bacteria.

Tea can lead to the inhibition of HIV. New research from the Journal of Allergy and Clinical Immunology has found that a substance found in green tea may inhibit the HIV virus from binding and can be a healthy part of a suppression regiment.

Tea may help prevent diabetes. There is some evidence to suggest that green tea helps lower the risk of getting Type 2 Diabetes, though future research is needed to confirm the association.

Tea can lower blood sugar. Tea contains catechin and polysaccharides which have been demonstrated to have a noticeable effect on lowering blood sugar.

Tea can prevent iron damage. Those suffering from iron disorders like haemochromatosis may be helped by drinking tea, which contains tannins that limit the amount of iron the body can absorb.

Tea can help with nasal decongestion. If you've got a bit of a cold, drinking black tea with lemon may help clear up some of the congestion that's bothering you. Just make sure your body doesn't become dependent on the treatment.

MORE GREAT HEALTH BENEFITS OF TEA

Anti-Cancer - Multiple studies have shown that the antioxidant compounds in tea have cancer fighting characteristics. Tea also provides inhibitory effects on DNA synthesis of leukemia cells and lung carcinoma cells. Tea has been linked to being both preventative and combative against many different types of cancer.

Anti-Heart Disease - Green tea has been shown to fight obesity and lower LDL "bad" cholesterol-two risk factors for heart disease and diabetes. Tea has also been shown to improve blood vessel function.

Anti-Stroke - Research presented at the International Stroke Conference in February 2009 found that drinking three or more cups of tea per day can reduce the risk of suffering a stroke by as much as 21%. The research, conducted at the University of California, Los Angeles, found that drinking green and black varieties of teas has a significant impact on the risk of stroke and cardiovascular disease.

Anti-Arthritis - Tea has been shown to provide rheumatoid arthritis prevention and relief.

Increased Mental Awareness - The amino acid L-theanine, which is found almost exclusively in the tea plant, affects the brain's neurotransmitters and increases alpha brain-wave activity. The result is a calmer, yet more alert, state of mind.

Weight Loss - In clinical trials conducted by the University of Geneva and the University of Birmingham it was found that tea raises metabolic rates, speeds up fat oxidation and improves insulin sensitivity. In addition, green tea contains catechin polyphenols that raise thermogenesis (the production of heat by the body), and hence increases fat expenditure.

Immune System - L-theanine may help the body's immune system response when fighting infection, by boosting the disease-fighting capacity of gamma delta T cells.

Lowered Stress Levels - Drinking black tea can lead to lower levels of the stress hormone cortisol. Blood platelet activation, which is linked to blood clotting and the risk of heart attacks has also been shown to be lower for tea drinkers.

Oral Health- Researchers at the University of Illinois, Chicago conducted a study which revealed that polyphenols found in tea help inhibit the growth of bacteria that cause bad breath, and can inhibit the creation of dental cavities.

Cardiovascular Health- Research has shown that black tea improves blood vessel reactivity, reducing both blood pressure and arterial stiffness, indicating better overall cardiovacular health.

Tea seems to be a natural and pleasant way to increase whole body health and well being, both mentally and physically. In addition to the studies conducted revealing the great health benefits of tea...the mere act of making a cup of tea... and sitting down to enjoy it, seems to have a profound effect on body, mind, and soul. This effect maybe isn't something best measured by science. Rather, it is just something that we feel.

CHAPTER 3:
14 DAY TEA CLEANSE PLAN

16 WAYS TO LOSE 15 POUNDS WITH TEA IN 14 DAYS

It describes an easy and effective protocol for stripping away belly fat fast, you don't necessarily have to follow it exactly. Here are some of the most effective hacks to use when you're ready to lose weight—at the sound of a whistle.

1 FOCUS ON GREEN TEA

Every tea has its own special weight-loss powers, but if your boat is sinking and you can only grab one package of tea before swimming to the deserted island, make it green tea. Green tea is the bandit that picks the lock on your fat cells and drains them away, even when we're not making the smartest dietary choices. Chinese researchers found that green tea significantly lowers triglyceride concentrations (potentially dangerous fat found in the blood) and belly fat in subjects who eat fatty diets. Follow these steps to Make the Perfect Cup of Green Tea!

2 MAKE IT YOUR POST-WORKOUT DRINK

Brazilian scientists found that participants who consumed three cups of the beverage every day for a week had fewer markers of the cell damage caused by resistance to exercise. That means that green tea can also help you recover faster after an intense workout. In another study—this one on people—participants who combined a daily habit of four to five cups of green tea each day with a 25-minute workout for 11 days lost an average of two more pounds than the non-tea-drinking exercisers.

3 UPGRADE TO MATCHA

The concentration of EGCG—the superpotent nutrient found in green tea—may be as much as 137 times greater in powdered matcha tea. EGCG can simultaneously boost lipolysis (the breakdown of fat) and block adipogenesis (the formation of new fat cells). One study found that men who drank green tea containing 136 milligrams of EGCG—what you'd find in a single 4-gram serving of matcha—lost twice as much weight than a placebo group and four times as much belly fat over the course of three months

4 PREGAME WITH TEA

Before you head out to dinner, pour yourself a cup of green tea. The active ingredient in green tea, EGCG, boosts levels of cholecystokinin, or CCK, a hunger-quelling hormone. In a Swedish study that looked at green tea's effect on hunger, researchers divided up participants into two groups: One group sipped water with their meal and the other group drank green tea. Not only did tea-sippers report less of a desire to eat their favorite foods (even two hours after sipping the brew), they found those foods to be less satisfying.

5 DRINK TEA RIGHT BEFORE BED

You probably already know that chamomile tea can help induce sleep (there's even a brand called Sleepy Time). But science is showing that teas actually work on a hormonal level to lower our agita and bring peace and slumber. Studies have found that herbal teas like valerian and hops contain compounds that can actually reduce levels of stress hormones in our bodies, bringing on sleep — and reducing the body's ability to store fat!

6 AND DRINK IT RIGHT WHEN YOU WAKE UP

A study in the International Journal of Molecular Science found that fasting overnight, followed by green tea intake (at least 30 minutes before your first meal of the day), allowed for the best possible absorption of EGCG, the magic nutrient in green tea.

7 DRINK RED WHEN YOU'RE SEEING RED

Red tea, also known as rooibos, is a great choice for when you're struggling with midday stress. What makes rooibos particularly good for soothing your mind is the unique flavanoid called Aspalathin. Research shows this compound can reduce stress hormones that trigger hunger and fat storage and are linked to hypertension, metabolic syndrome, cardiovascular disease, insulin resistance and type 2 diabetes.

8 MEET A FRIEND FOR TEA

A new study in the journal Hormones and Behavior found that those who feel lonely experience greater circulating levels of the appetite-stimulating hormone ghrelin after they eat, causing them to feel hungrier sooner. Over time, folks who are perennially lonely simply take in more calories than those with stronger social support networks.

9 KEEP IT IN THE DARK

The active ingredients in teas are highly unstable under sunlight. Keep tea in a dark, dry place. Storing tea in sealed packaging in cool, dark conditions helps increase shelf life. If you brew iced tea, it will stay good for about 4 days, as long as you keep it refrigerated.

10 MAKE A FAT-MELTING DRESSING

To add the power of green tea's catechins on top, steep tea bags in oils (or vinegars) to create richly flavored salad dressings. A study in Nutrition Journal found that those who ate monounsaturated fats at lunch reported a 40 percent decreased desire to eat for hours afterward. Check out these Delicious Recipes Using Matcha Green Tea!

11 BLEND IT INTO A SMOOTHIE

Green or white teas make great bases for smoothies. In a study presented at the North American Association of the Study of Obesity, researchers found that regularly drinking smoothies in place of meals increased a person's chances of losing weight and keeping it off longer than a year. Add your favorite tea to one of these 56 Smoothie Recipes for Weight Loss!

12 TOSS IN SOME CHIA SEEDS

These little black morsels of nutrition are packed with fiber, protein and, most important of all, omega-3 fatty acids. Pair chia seeds with green tea in a smoothie to turbocharge the tea's fat-burning powers. According to a study review in the International Journal of Molecular Science, omega-3 polyunsaturated fatty acids may enhance not only the bioavailability of EGCG, but also its effectiveness.

13 COOK YOUR OATMEAL IN IT

Why not empower rice, quinoa and even oatmeal with the belly-fat burning properties of green tea? Tie 4 green tea bags onto a wooden spoon. Fill a small pot with 2 cups water; add wooden spoon and tea bags. Bring water to a boil and remove tea bags. Add the grains to the boiling tea water and cook as directed. Try it with these delicious Quinoa Recipes for Weight Loss!

14 PEPPER UP YOUR MEALS

When you drink tea with a salad or soup, make an effort to add some black pepper to your meal. Recent studies have indicated that a compound found in black pepper, called piperine, may help improve blood levels of EGCG by allowing it to linger in the digestive system longer — meaning that more of it is absorbed by the body.

15 MAKE A MATCHA PARFAIT

Yogurt is a great weight-loss food — until you start adding flavoring to it. Fruit-on-the-bottom teas can have as many sugar calories as a candy bar. For a fast boost of flavor, stir matcha powder into plain, full-fat Greek yogurt. Try it with one of these 25 Best Yogurts for Weight Loss!

16 TURN LEFTOVERS INTO SUPERFOODS

Ochazuke is a quickie foodie trick from Japan. It's made by pouring a cup of hot green tea over a bowl of leftover rice, then topping the bowl with savory ingredients to create a terrific slim-down lunch. Place the rice in a bowl. Pour the hot tea over it. Top with crackers, flaked salmon, seaweed, lime juice and soy sauce.

CHAPTER 4:
16 DELICIOUS TEA RECIPES

STEP REFRIGERATOR TEA
- 4 tea bags
- 4 cups water
  Fill a pitcher or mason jar with water. Hang tea bags in the water. Cover and steep 6-12 hours in the refrigerator. Serve as desired with any flavorings or sweeteners.

CHEAP AND EASY FLAVORED TEA RECIPE
- 3 family sized tea bags
- 4 flavored tea bags (lemon, blueberry, blackberry, mint, orange, cinnamon– Any flavor will work.)
- 1 cup sugar
  Pour 4 cups boiling water over the tea bags and allow to steep for 6 minutes. Remove and squeeze the tea bags. Add sugar and stir until dissolved. Pour into a gallon pitcher and add cold water and ice to fill.

BLUEBERRY TEA RECIPE
- 1 (16-oz.) pkg. blueberries (frozen or fresh)
- 1/2 cup lemon juice
- 4 cups water
- 4 cups brewed tea
- 3/4 cup sugar
  Bring the blueberries and lemon juice to a boil in a large saucepan over medium heat. Cook, stirring occasionally, for 5 minutes. Remove from the heat and pour through a fine wire-mesh strainer into a bowl, using

the back of a spoon to squeeze out the juice. You can freeze the solids in ice cube trays and use for smoothies. Stir 3/4 cup sugar and the blueberry juice mixture into the tea. Pour into a pitcher. Cover and chill 1 hour. Serve over ice. Makes 4 servings.

RASPBERRY TEA RECIPE

- 1 (16-oz.) pkg. raspberries (frozen or fresh)
- 4 cups water
- 3/4 cup sugar
- 4 cups brewed tea
  Bring the raspberries and water to a boil in a large saucepan over medium heat. Cook, stirring occasionally, for 5 minutes. Remove from the heat and pour through a fine wire-mesh strainer into a bowl, using the back of a spoon to squeeze out the juice. Add the tea to a pitcher. Stir in the sugar and raspberry juice mixture. Chill 1 hour. Serve over ice.

COPYCAT OLIVE GARDEN PEACH TEA RECIPE

- 1 cup sugar
- 1 cup water
- 2-3 sliced fresh peaches
- 6 cups brewed tea
  Place the sugar, 1 cup of the water and the peaches into a saucepan and cook until they come to a boil. Reduce the heat to a simmer (medium). Crush the peaches as you stir to dissolve the sugar. Once the sugar is dissolved, turn off the burner, cover, and allow the mixture to rest for about 30 minutes. Strain the syrup to remove the fruit pieces. Save the fruit pieces for smoothies. Add the syrup to the tea and refrigerate. Serve over ice.

ORANGE TEA RECIPE

- 2-3 cups brewed tea, still hot
- 1 cup sugar
- 1 orange, sliced
- 1 tsp. vanilla

- Dash cinnamon

  Place the oranges in the bottom of a pitcher. Add vanilla and cinnamon. Pour the tea into the pitcher while still hot so the sugar dissolves and top off with water. Serve over ice.

STRAWBERRY ICED TEA RECIPE

- 3 cups brewed tea
- 4 cups fresh or frozen strawberries
- 1 1/2 cups water
- 1 1/2 cups sugar (or sweetener of your choice)

  In a saucepan, boil the strawberries, sugar, and water. Lower the heat and simmer for 10-15 minutes. Cool slightly. Pour the syrup through a fine mesh sieve into a gallon pitcher. You can freeze the solids in ice cube trays and use for smoothies.

  Pour the tea into the pitcher with the syrup and stir. Fill the pitcher with cold water. Chill completely. Then serve over ice and/or freshly frozen strawberries.

EASY PEACH TEA RECIPE

- 8 cups brewed tea
- 3/4 cup sugar
- 11-ounce can peach nectar (found in the fruit juice section or alcoholic drink section)

  In a 10-12 cup pitcher, pour the ingredients and stir until the sugar is dissolved. Add ice until the pitcher is full. Serve.

MINT LIME TEA COOLER

- 4 cups brewed tea
- 1 1/2 cups sugar
- Juice from 6 limes
- Fresh mint or raspberries for a flavor twist and cute garnish

  Add the sugar to a one gallon pitcher. Add the brewed tea. Add enough water to equal one gallon of tea. Add the lime juice and a few mint sprigs. Stir until the sugar is dissolved. Serve over ice and garnish with mint sprigs if desired. This mint lime tea is best served cold with ice!

JOLLY RANCHER TEA RECIPE

- 1 tea bag
- 4 Jolly Ranchers, any flavor
  Brew the tea and Jolly Ranchers in boiling water. Serve hot or cold over ice.

CITRUS TEA RECIPE

- 6 cups water
- 2 regular individual sized tea bags
- 6 Tbsp. honey or sugar
- 1 stick cinnamon (which gives it just the right amount of zing)
- Juice of 2 lemons
- Slices of orange, lemon, lime and/or cucumber.
  Bring the water to a boil in a large saucepan, with cinnamon and sugar. Remove from the heat and drop in the tea bags. Cover and let it rest for 1 hour. Pour the tea into a pitcher, discarding the cinnamon stick. Stir in lemon juice. Add sliced fruits. Refrigerate overnight or until chilled. Add ice cubes and slices of citrus before serving.

BLACKBERRY TEA RECIPE

- 5 regular sized tea bags
- 4 cups boiling water
- 1/4 cup mint leaves, crushed
- 1/2 cup sugar
- 2 lbs. blackberries
  Brew the tea and mint in boiling water. Strain. Stir in the sugar. Purée the blackberries in a blender or food processor. Strain through a fine sieve. Discard the pulp and seeds. Stir the blackberry purée into the tea.

  Taste and adjust the sugar as desired. Chill. Serve over ice garnished with mint leaf and 2 or 3 blackberries.

TROPICAL ORANGE TEA RECIPE

- 6 cups refrigerator tea
- 1 2/3 cups pineapple juice
- Juice from 1 large lemon
- Juice from 1 large orange
- 1 cup sugar

Pour the tea into a pitcher. Add the pineapple juice, lemon juice, orange juice and sugar. Stir to combine. Chill the tea until you're ready to serve.

BOSTON ICED TEA

INGREDIENTS:

- 2 liters water
- 1/2 cup white sugar
- 8 tea bags (black tea)
- 2 cups cranberry juice concentrate

DIRECTIONS:

In a medium-sized pan or pot, bring the water to a boil. Add sugar and stir until dissolved. Remove from heat. Allow to cool for 1-2 minutes. Add teabags and steep for 5 minutes or until desired strength is achieved. Stir in cranberry juice concentrate. Allow to cool for 5-10 minutes before placing in the refrigerator. Add ice cubes before serving.

ORANGE EARL GREY TEA

INGREDIENTS:

- 2 liters water
- 1/4 cup sugar
- 8 tea bags (Earl Grey Tea)
- 1 cup fresh orange juice
- 2 tablespoons sliced orange peels or peel of one orange

DIRECTIONS:

In a small pan, bring 1 liter of water to a boil. Stir in sugar until fully dissolved. Remove from heat. Allow to cool for 2 minutes. Steep the teabags and orange peels for 5 minutes or until desired strength is achieved. Remove the teabags and strain the orange peels. Place on a large pitcher. Add orange juice and 1 liter of cold water. Stir. Allow cooling for 5-10 minutes before placing in the refrigerator. Add ice cubes before serving.

HONEY-LEMON ICED GREEN TEA

INGREDIENTS:

- 2 liters water
- 2 cups honey
- 8 teabags (green tea)
- 1 medium-sized lemon ,

DIRECTIONS:

In a small pan or pot, bring to a boil 1 liter of water. Remove from heat and allow cooling for 3 minutes. Steep the teabags for 3 minutes or until desired strength is achieved. Remove teabags. Stir in honey. Add 1 liter of water and stir. Slice lemon into thin wedges and add to mixture. Allow to cool before placing in the refrigerator. Add ice cubes prior to serving.

Place slices of lemon or orange on the rim of the glass. Fill the glass with ice cubes before pouring the ice tea mixture.

If you are preparing this drink for a dinner party one way to really knock it out of the park, and provide the perfect chilled rink is to put the tea in the fridge to let it cool. Then about half an hour before your party begins put the pitcher in the freezer. This will bring down the core temperature and will ensure that the ice cubes don't melt right away. This avoids watering down your drink, while still having a cold beverage ready for your guests!

CHAPTER 5:
THE DO'S AND DON'TS ON A TEA CLEANSE

WHAT IS A TEATOX?

A teatox is a detox using tea. You detox by drinking specially formulated tea to cleanse the body.

Tea uses a blend of all-natural herbal ingredients, carefully selected, sourced, blended and expertly formulated to help maximize your body's detox ability and kick-start a healthy lifestyle.

DOS

Consult your doctor before teatoxing if you have a pre-existing medical condition

If you are under 15 years of age, you should discuss with your parents whether teatoxing is right for you

To be on the safe side, do take the pill in the morning after you have been to the toilet and had your breakfast or early in the evening, 2-3 hours before you take the Night Cleanse Tea. Please do check with your doctor if you have any doubt.

DON'TS

Teatox is not a meal-replacement program so eat regularly and don't skip meals

Do not take our tea if you are pregnant or breastfeeding as our blends are too strong for babies

Morning Boost shouldn't be drunk after 5pm as the caffeine may interfere with your sleep

Do not drink Night Cleanse tea during fasting periods as it might result in watery stools, as there is no solid food to flush out. There is also limited water intake during fasting and drinking the tea might result in further dehydration.